I Became Your Mama

written by

MOLLIE HUYCK

illustrations by ÉMILIE FLEURY

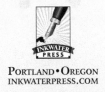

INKWATER PRESS

PORTLAND • OREGON
INKWATERPRESS.COM

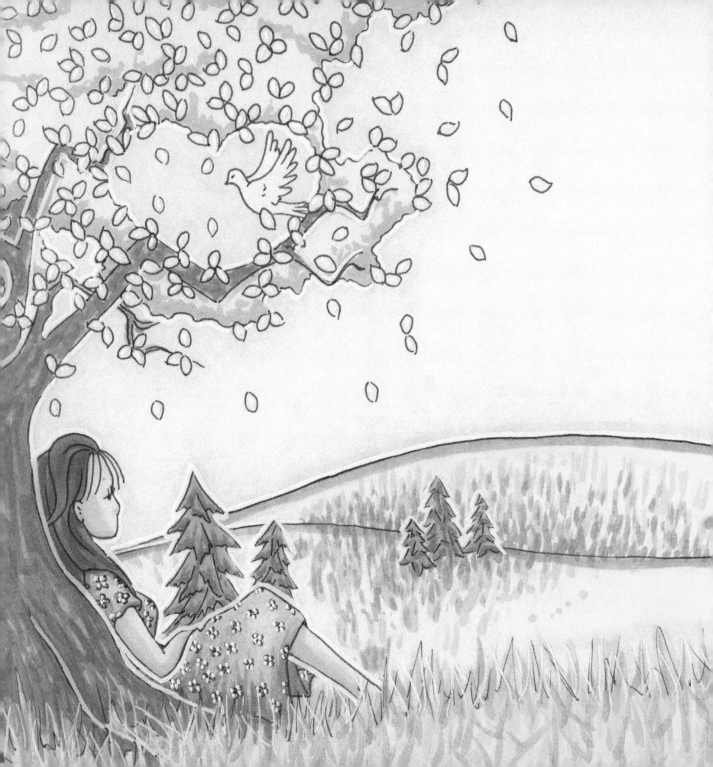

I've dreamt of you forever.
I love you so much.

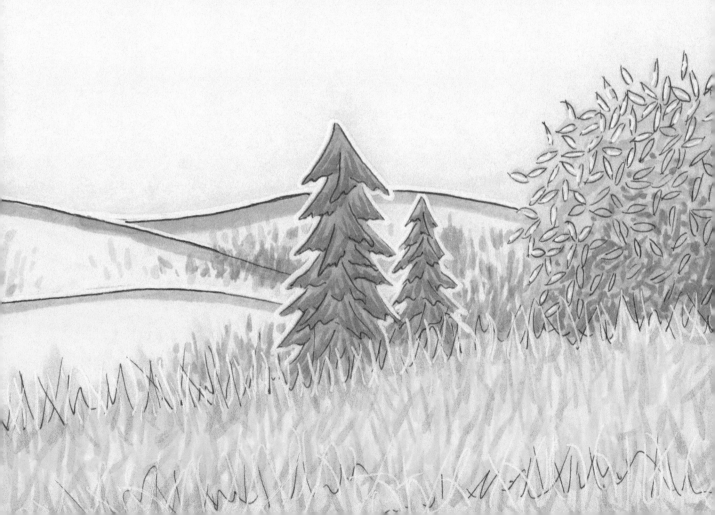

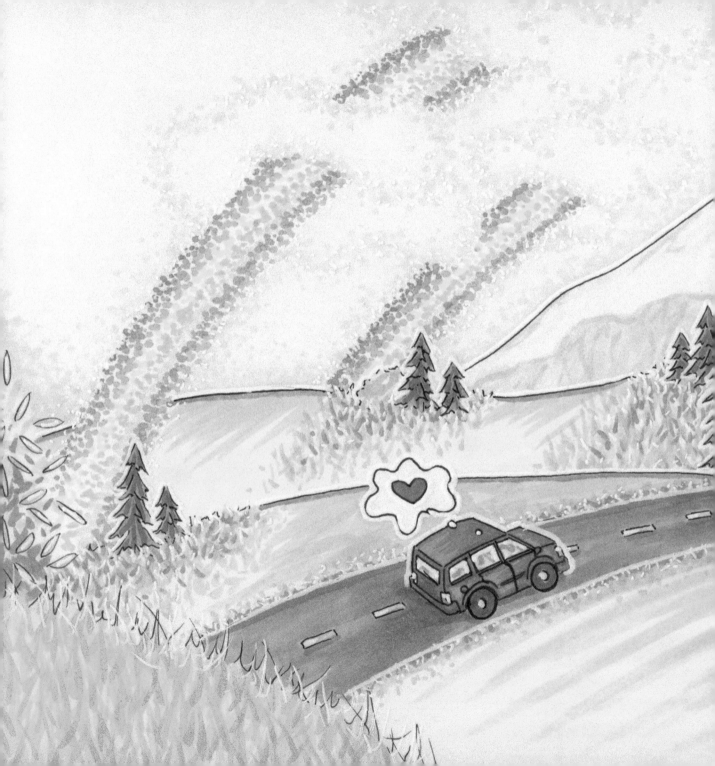

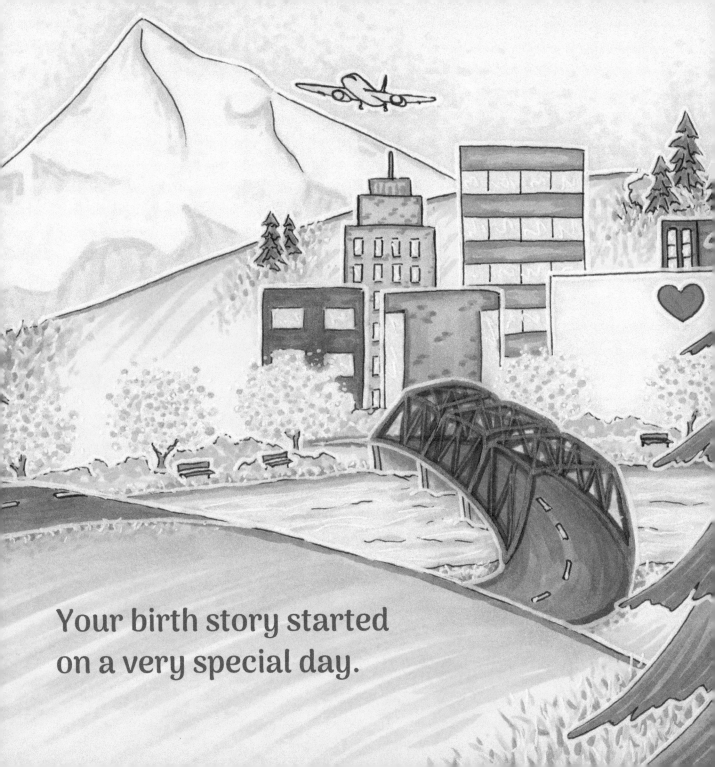

Your birth story started
on a very special day.

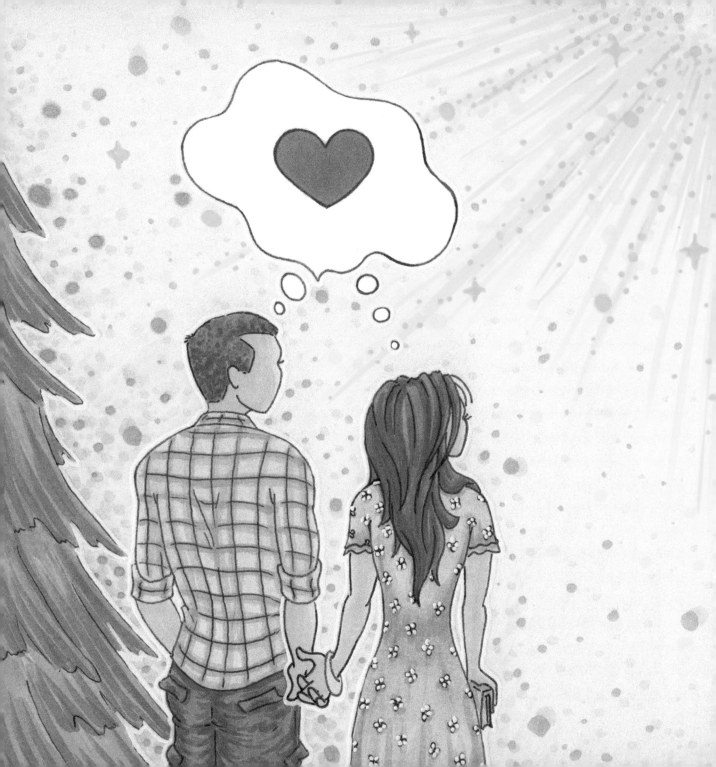

With love, faith, and science,
you grew in a wonderful way.

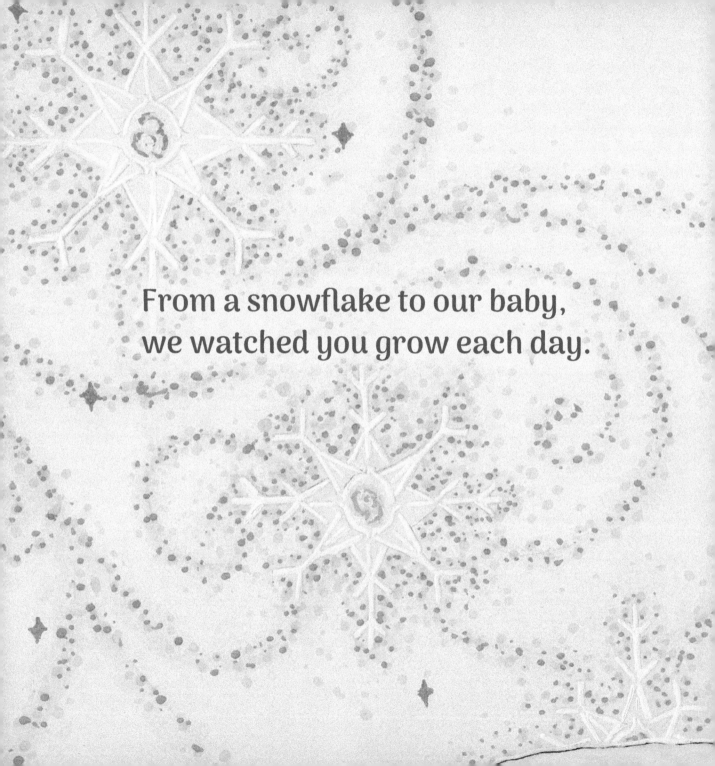

From a snowflake to our baby,
we watched you grow each day.

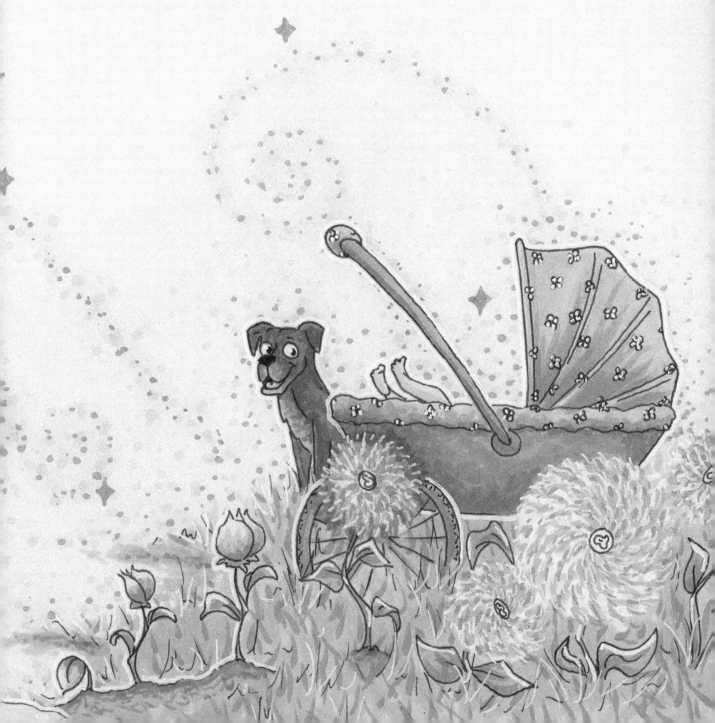

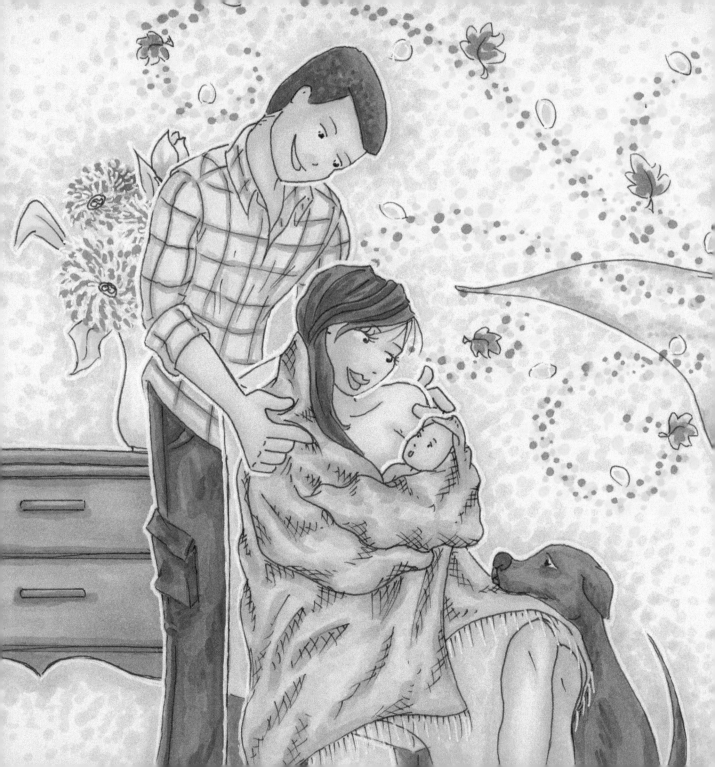

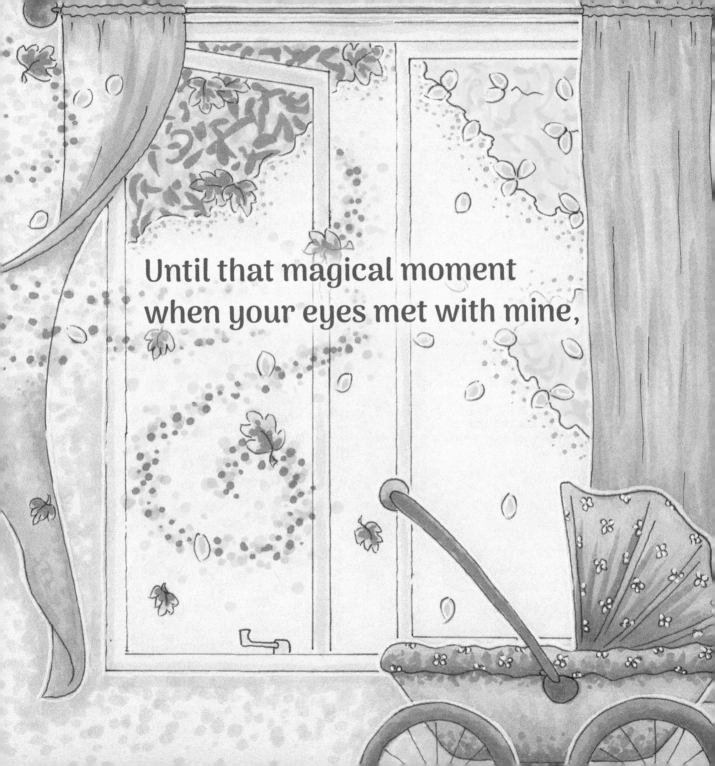

Until that magical moment
when your eyes met with mine,

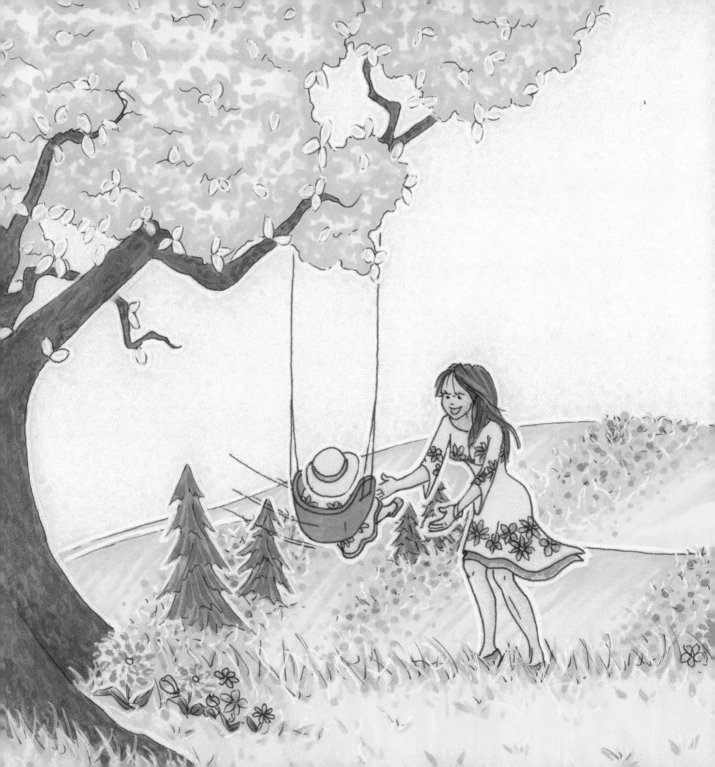

I became your mama,
and forever you'll be mine.

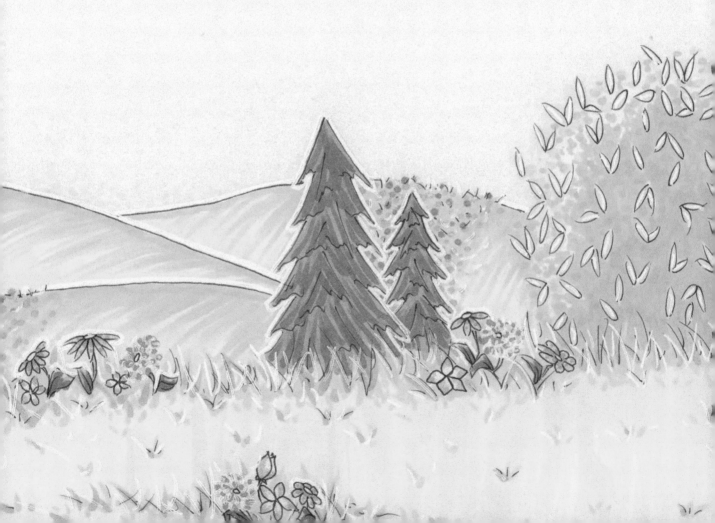

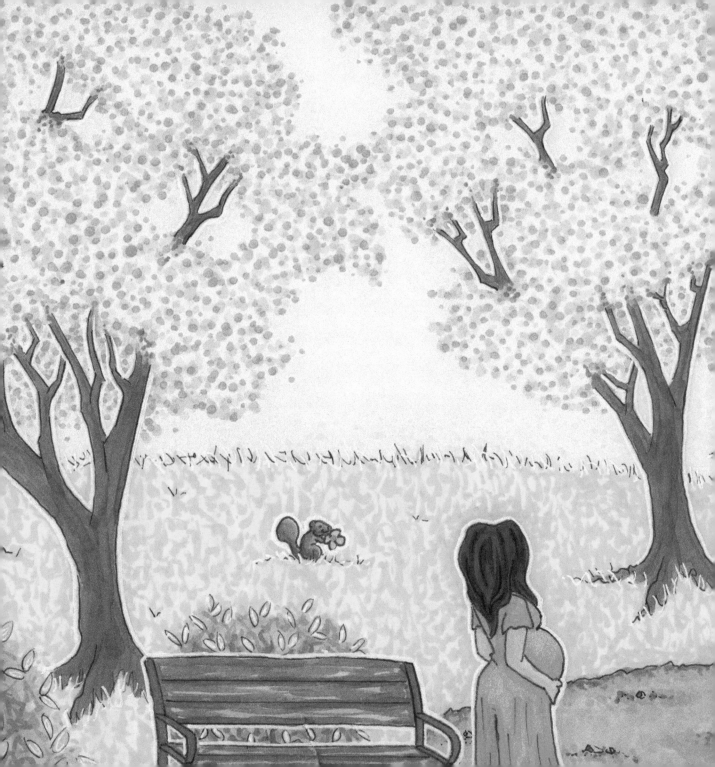

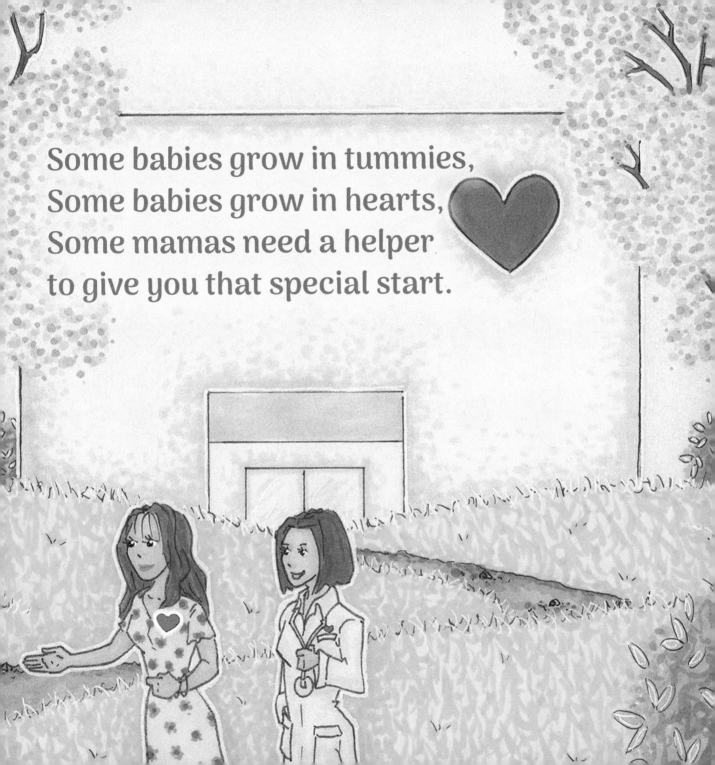

Some babies grow in tummies,
Some babies grow in hearts,
Some mamas need a helper
to give you that special start.

But no matter how you grew,
know that you are wanted, loved, and true.

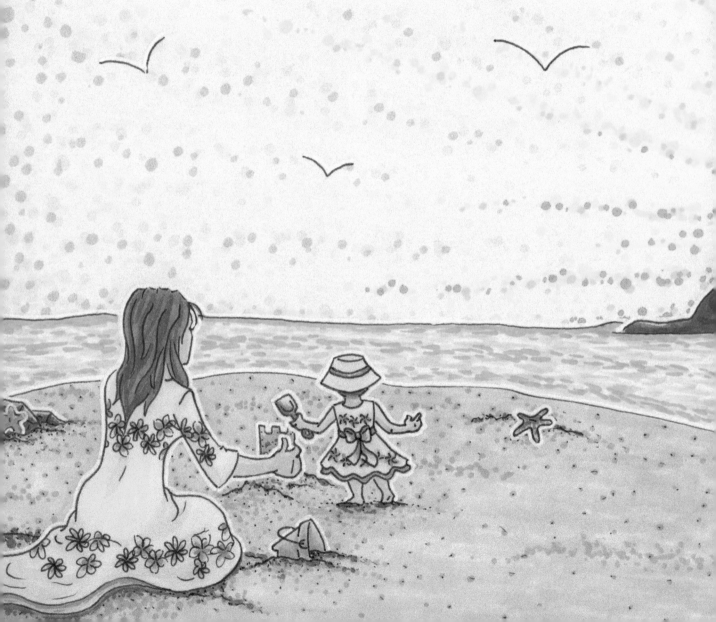

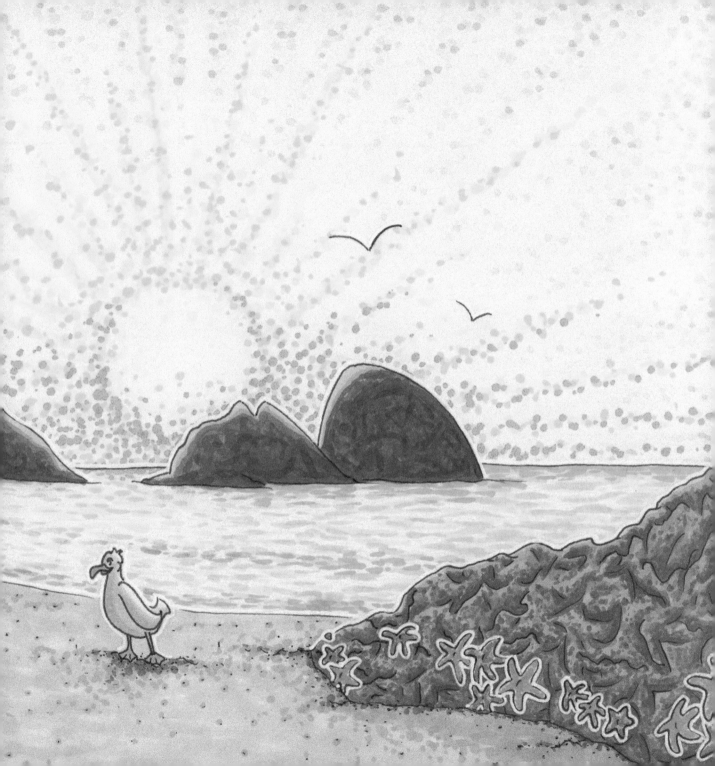

For My Daughter

CPSIA information can be obtained
at www.ICGtesting.com
Printed in the USA
LVHW071450231118
598057LV00015B/293/P